# What are you Looking at?

Erin Wakeland

What are you Looking at?

Copyright© 2021 by Erin Wakeland

Fifth Avenue Press is a locally focused and publicly owned publishing imprint of the Ann Arbor District Library. It is dedicated to supporting the local writing community by promoting the production of original fiction, non-fiction and poetry written for children, teens and adults.

Printed in the United States of America

First Printing, 2021

ISBN: Paperback: 9781947989894; Ebook: 9781947989900

Fifth Avenue Press

343 S Fifth Ave

Ann Arbor, MI 48104

fifthavenue.press

Editing

Ann Arbor District Library

Layout and Design

Erin Wakeland

Returning Red Solo      8

You Have Everything You Need      42

The Postcard Experiment      90

Artist-in-Residence      118

# Introduction

I spent my days as a college student furiously biking from class to waiting tables at a French restaurant, photographing student music shows, picking up shifts at the flower shop, and returning home to projects sprawled across the room. An object in motion will stay in motion, and I was soaring. The adrenaline of doing things carried me through worries about post-grad, self-worth, and what it all means to be here. Busyness was my vice.

A switch flipped when I received critical reviews on a project my sophomore year. I realized that more work didn't equate to better work. Speeding through the process of achieving your goals is like fast-forwarding a movie: brief and cheated of pleasure. I took the summer off. I thought of myself, or lack of self, as I worked on an archaeological site in Rome, Italy. I felt no pressure for what I was doing to mean anything for the greater me. I was there to observe things that I had no expertise on. I had no idea what people were saying around me. I dug in the dirt, I cleaned pottery, I ate gelato and I did nothing to self-improve.

My research is experiential: I learn by doing, by conversing with friends, by going for long walks, by attempting my hand at doing nothing. I untangled my ideas of self-worth from productivity according to the capitalist value system, or should I say: I'm continuously trying to. I still find myself in the throes of productivity culture, and the best way I can detect overload is to observe where my attention is when I'm crossing the street, when I'm riding the bus, when I'm listening to a lecture. Through this project, I try to recover my everyday life from the culturally present commodification of time and self-hood for profit: the definition I give capitalism throughout this project.

I seek to explore the relationships between worthiness, ordinariness, and what happens to people's attention in a capitalist system. To engage my ideas with everyday life, I re-framed activities like shopping, attending college, and throwing trash away through a series of public, performance-based social experiments. I completed four social experiments throughout my senior year. The final form is this book (hello!) that frames each experiment within a personal essay used to unpack my relationship to the topics at hand. The book includes a variety of media used to document each scenario through photography, painting, and inter-views. Ultimately, *What are you Looking at?* offers insight into the hardships of utilizing one's attention to redefine what it means to live well while steeped in American capitalist culture.

### I woke up today in the same house

I've been waking up in for two years. The creak of the stairs is my morning hymn as I totter down to brew coffee. My house is old. It was built in 1906 and has poor insulation to prove it. Surrounding it are typical college houses, apartments, and fraternities crammed together like LEGO pieces.

I wonder what the street looked like in 1906: a dirt road patterned with the shadows of trees, a few idle horses, and a good view of the cemetery two blocks away. Certainly shoes were not hanging from telephone wires, nor were makeshift beer-pong tables splayed out like smashed bugs in yards, trash blowing down gutters like tumbleweed.

It is October in the South University neighborhood of Ann Arbor, Michigan. To get home, I walk past the Theta Chi fraternity house. I am well informed of this fraternity's doings through locational osmosis (I'm often awoken on Saturday mornings by their blaring of Mr. Brightside by the Killers).

The artifacts left on the sidewalks and yards are not uncommon across the neighborhood, but Theta Chi is the biggest culprit of littering on my street. I've collected some beautifully smashed cans that now hang in my studio. The red solo cup, a frat party emblem, remains aplenty across their yard and spills into the gutter.

Map of what my local geography feels like:

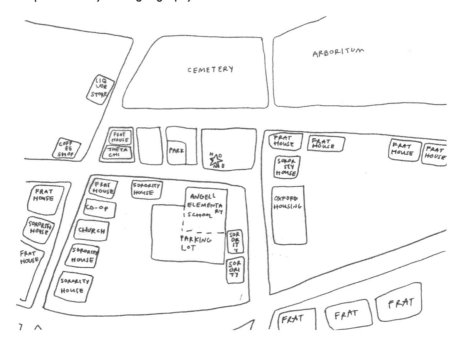

**Actual map:**

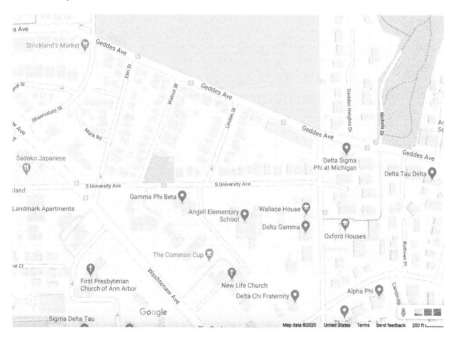

These little red sirens tease me on my walk home, luring me with their song of a micro-plastic free water source if I pick them up. They peek through matted leaves and dirty snow caps like rubies, the broken ones still traceable to their original form.

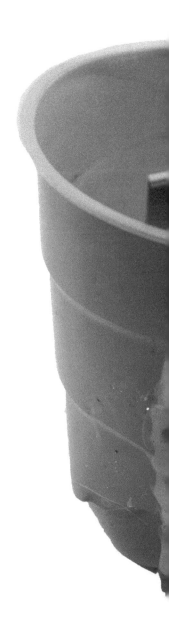

I walk by these cups and think about a reality in which they are as precious as rubies. We would keep our cup at the party and wash it out when we are finished. We would stack it with the glass cups or position it like a trophy in the display of chinaware. When it breaks we would repair it. When it is beyond repair we would still treasure it.

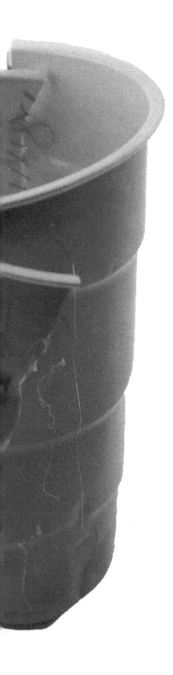

I experiment with how long I can take my packed lunch in the plastic bag that once held sandwich bread before it tears. I ran out of maple syrup and use the bottle to hold salad dressing. I made a sweater out of a thrifted blanket and patch my jeans when they tear.

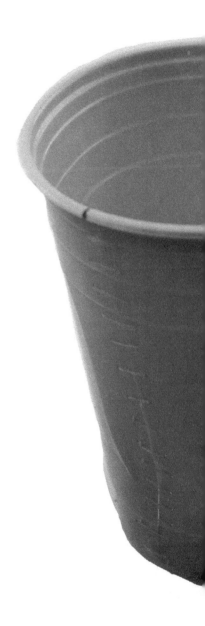

In my own life, I try to smooth out the hierarchy of preciousness that I assign to the objects surrounding me. By doing so I hope to pay closer attention to what I consume and become imaginative with how I use things.

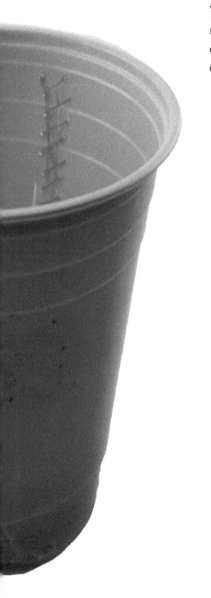

The life of the red solo cup post-drink is currently unaccounted for: what if we treated the cup with the same integrity as an object with emotional and monetary worth?

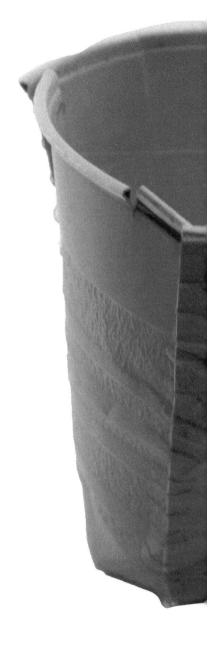

I started to collect the strewn cups outside
the Theta Chi fraternity house on the corner
of Washtenaw Ave and South University Ave.
In the evening, I tediously mended them like
it was 1906 and I was waiting for the fire to
burnout while Pa played the fiddle.

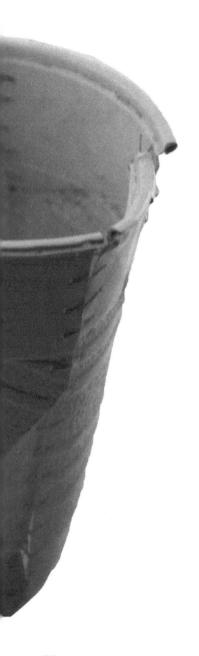

I needle-punched holes parallel to the cracks of the cup and laced the red thread through. Sometimes the holes would split leaving me with more work to do. Once, absolutely frustrated with the pace of this activity, I tried to hot glue a crack. It bubbled and singed holes through the red, thin plastic. Too hot. I began to question everything. Treat it preciously, I repeated in my head, holding myself to my intention. I picked up the needle again.

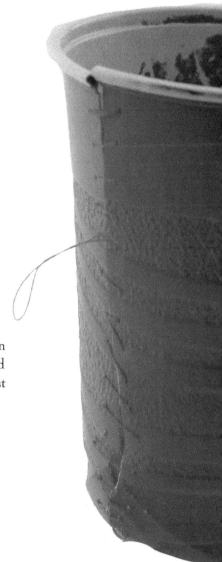

Despite my care in mending them, you can spot my cups in a lineup. They are clumsy and odd and certainly not suave. Nevertheless, last Saturday afternoon, during the Theta Chi party for the Penn State vs. University of Michigan game, I ventured over to their backyard tailgate to return their possessions. Videographer Miriam Siegel followed me to document the interactions.

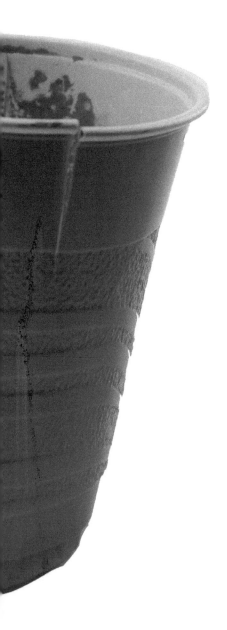

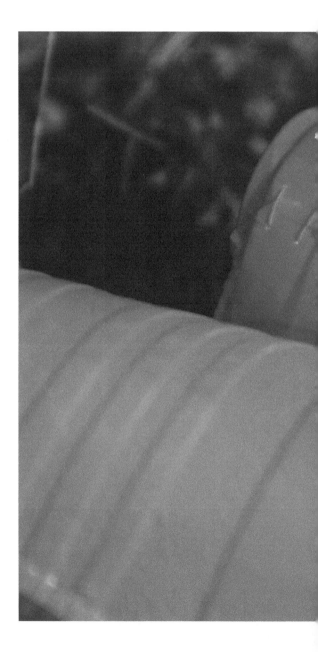

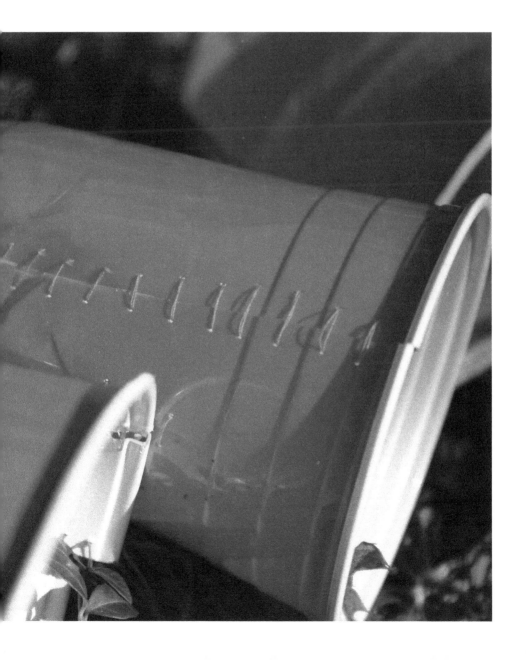

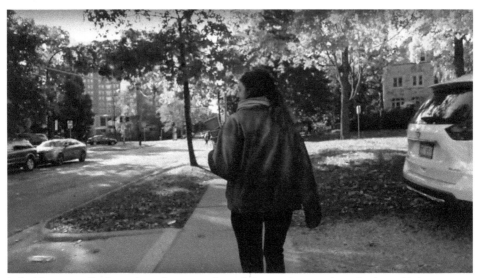

I decide to try the front door first even though I see where to hop the knee-high gate partitioning off the party in the backyard.

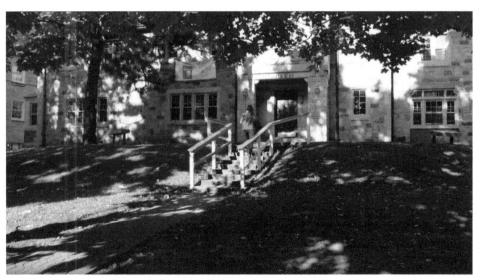

I'm cordial, I'm neighborly; I'll abide by formalities.

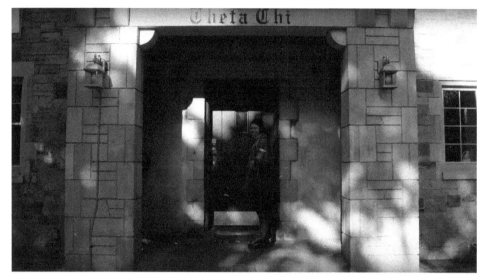

Many knocks later I doubt there is a doorman tending to solicitors.

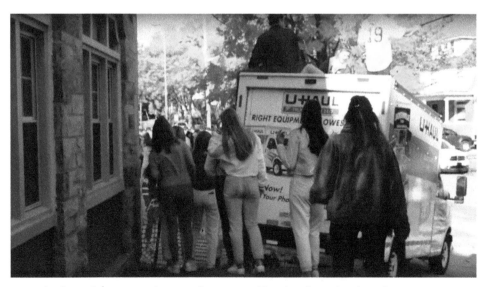

I join the fence-hoppers in the rite of passage. Shortly after, I land my first interaction.

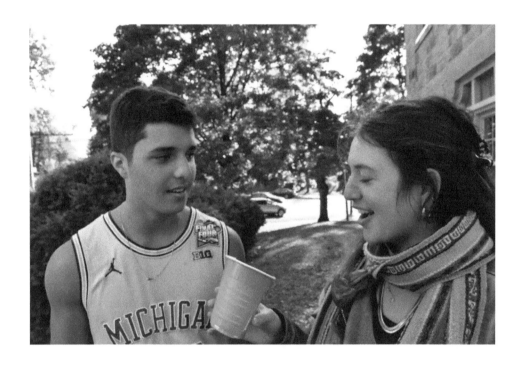

**EW:** Hi, are you in a frat?
(A major oversight was not asking for names so I will resort to diminutive cast names.)

**Party Boy #1:** Yes, ADPi.

**EW:** Oh so not this one?

**Party Boy #1:** No not this one.

**EW:** Well, I found these cups in this yard and I fixed them so you can use them again at your parties. Would you use them?

**Party Boy #1:** No they are too dirty.
*Hands him another cup*

**EW:** How about this one?

**Party Boy #1:** Dirty also. Why did you fix them?

**EW:** Because someone left them in the yard and —

**Party Boy #1:** I can recycle them?

**EW:** Yeah, well you can reuse them.
*Picks another mended cup*

**Party Boy #1:** I would drink out of this cup.

**EW:** Okay. Do you want to drink from it now?

**Party Boy #1:** No not right now but in the future.

**EW:** Okay.

**Miriam, behind the videotape interrupts:** Will you take better care of the cups now?

**Party Boy #1:** Now that it is sewed, I'll definitely take better care of it. People want a recycling bin at parties.

**EW:** That would be great. Would you do it?

**Party Boy #1:** Yes, for sure. We don't have anywhere to throw out our cups.

**EW:** Where do you put them now?

**Party Boy #1:** On the floor, in the garbage can, on the street. We liter them, it's terrible. If we had a recycling bin and put a red cup logo on there people would love it.

**EW:** You should bring that to the board.

**Party Boy #1:** I'm on the board.

**EW:** Oh so you have the power to change that.

**Party Boy #1:** I got it. I'll do it for you guys.
I was surprised by his effort to say exactly what he thought

I wanted to hear. I wasn't trying to tell people
to recycle. And I don't think I hit the objec-
tive of instilling a communist view on object
importance during this conversation. Whether
or not some of his sincerity was cheeky, I hope
he remembers this conversation during his next
board meeting and goes for the red solo cup
receptacle idea.

Miriam and I walk further into the yard.
Other people's elbows knead my arms as the
ground gets sandier. Music, cheering, and loud
conversations ping pong through the crowd.
On the party's periphery, we land on our next
two subjects.

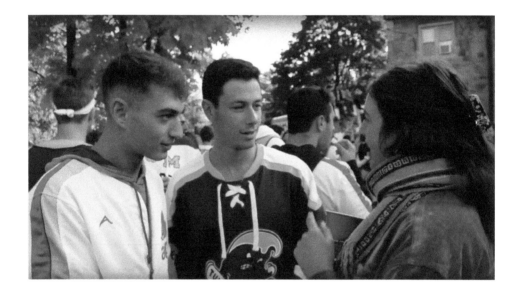

**EW:** Hey, are you both in a frat?

**Party Boy #2:** Yeah, but another one, not this one.

**EW:** Okay, that's alright. I found these cups outside this frat after a party last weekend and I fixed them up to use again.

**Party Boy #2:** Yeah, of course!
*Stares down into the cup like a water well*
It's pretty dirty though.
I don't know how I'd drink out of it now.

**Party Boy #3:** I feel like your drink would fall out.

**Party Boy #2:** Yeah it would spew.

**Party Boy #3:** Yeah maybe if you took a blow torch and did this: *motions up and down along a vertical crack in the cup*

**Party Boy #2:** I think we're getting poisoned. That's glue! *points to the glue holding another crack together on another cup*

We laugh a bit about how fragile the cups are. It's hard to play ignorant about the practicality of re-using the cups. But I also feel a timid attachment to the cup with the lumpy glue, like how you love your child even if they grow a gnarly wart on their big toe.

**EW:** Can you think of using these for another purpose?

**Them:** No not if you can't drink from them.

And I just like that I reached the limits of their imaginations.

I don't mean to brag, but at this point, I'm a bit of a spectacle. A small line gathers around me waiting to see these cups. I clutch my cups harder. Heads peer in and out of the semi-circle I've made with the next three sub-jects. Above us, vape clouds blow like the trade winds.

**EW:** Hi! Are you all in Greek life?

**Girl in Stripes:** Yes!

**Girl in Tie-Dye:** Yes!

**Boy with Sunglasses:** Ya!

**EW:** I fixed these cups up after I found them in the yard of this Frat last weekend. Would you like to use one?

**Girl in Stripes responds firmly:** YES. I'll pour my drink into it right now.

Boy with Sunglasses examines the cups very particularly. Girl in Stripes pours sprite into the cup. It holds for a few seconds and drips out.

**Boy with Sunglasses:** Yeah, that can't hold up.

We all disperse. Girl in Stripes took her cup with her as she greeted a friend nearby. I wave goodbye to her, but really it was to the cup. Life of the party, cup, you really were a star.

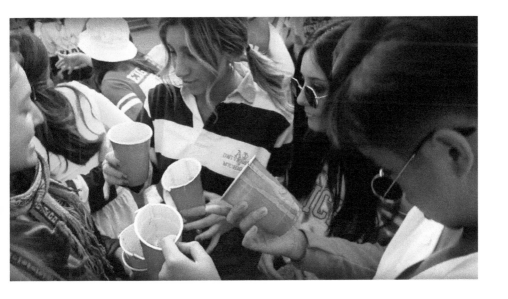

The gawkers ebb and flow with increasingly short attention spans. The music has gotten invasive as the bass is seriously disrupting our audio recording. My time is up, as I, distinct in my pink coat against the maize and blue, am stopped by a frat boy and asked to stop videoing. I could've stuck around, sipped a few beers and then sat on top of a U-Haul truck with the boys, but I decide to turn in.

I place the remaining cups in a storage cupboard next to the other plastic cups and the pile for spoons that accidentally fall into the garbage disposal. I don't have it in me to toss them into the recycling bin nor do I feel obliged to use them, but they remain precious to me.

I fought upstream to win others over in the
moments shared with the cups: they were spe-
cial for awhile, held by many hands, inspected
by curious eyes. The cups will stick together
pondering the outcome of the one snatched by
Girl in Stripes.

Maybe that cup is on a dorm room shelf,
iconic in suite 23, winning Girl in Stripes
strangest thing collected at a party. The other
cups will come out for the occasional party,
maybe my roommates will accidentally serve
sangria in them. But mostly, they will sit like
unearthed rubies in my dark cupboard. Their
brief glory days have passed, but ironically
they will outlive me after all. ∎

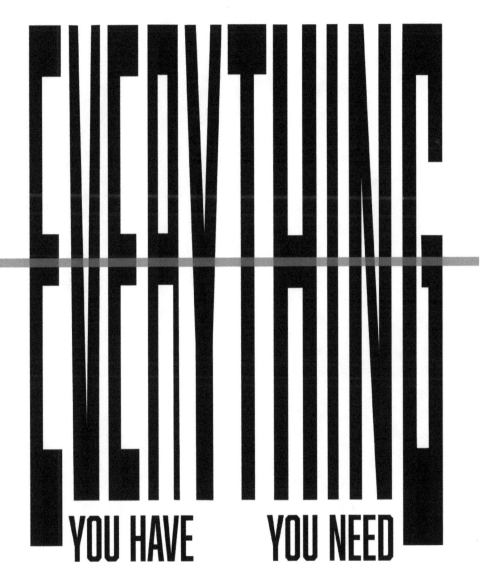

EVERYTHING

EVERYTHING

YOU HAVE     YOU NEED

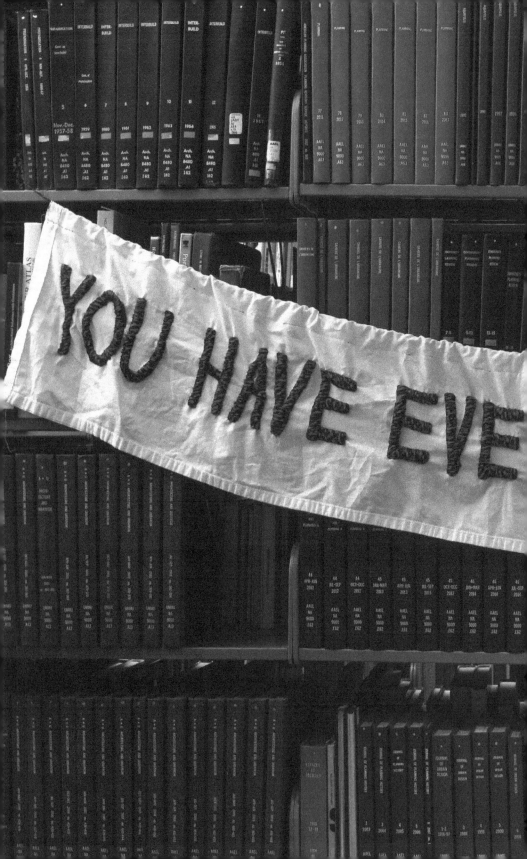

### Last spring, my professor Phoebe

Gloeckner told me to stop reading. I was making paintings based on the theory that text and image are interchangeable, and cornered her for a meeting on what to do next. I studied contemporary art like math equations; I was certain that if I could calculate the correct ratios I'd be the next Anselm Kiefer.

Phoebe gave me a puzzled look. And then suddenly at ease, she said "you already know everything you need to move forward, it's time to think about what you yourself think."

Research was my elegant form of procrastination, preventing me from moving forward, making things, and messing up. I was circling the library like a fish in its bowl, trying to perfectly calculate my next move as to prevent mistakes.

Is it possible to over-consume research the
way that we over-consume material things?

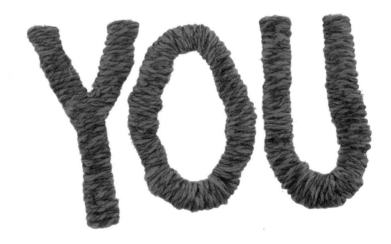

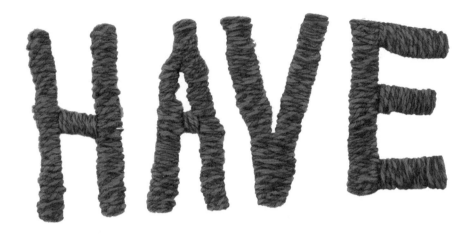

Maybe the consequences look different: it isn't that your wallet gets skinnier while your closet doors bust open, but perhaps the imbalance leaves you incapable of attending to others things in your life. Have I missed the point of making work with my head stuck in a book? If these words are true of this project, are they true for the rest of my life?

I decided to make a banner out of an old bed sheet and yarn to remind myself that I have everything I need. I thought a handmade banner was a perfect way to offset wants and desires: its presence is large and bold, but upon closer look, the uneven stitches and wiggly spaces reveal imperfection. Hopefully my message will get across with loving enthusiasm. I took the banner to the entrance of my favorite wing in the Art and Architecture library to investigate, to see if I could convince myself that I have everything I need.

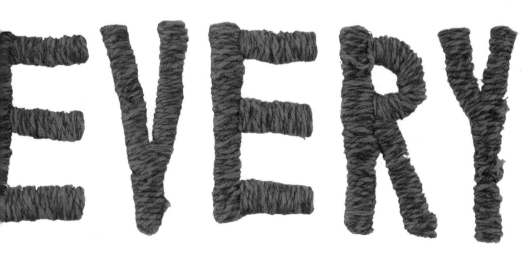

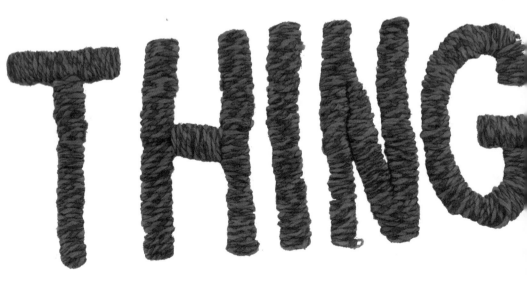

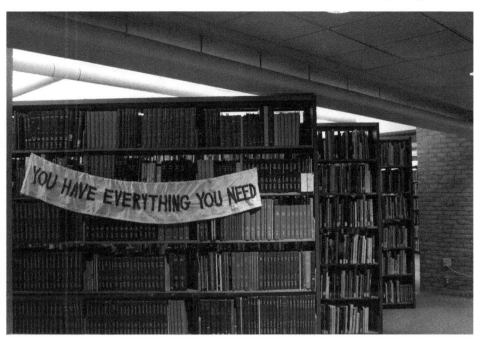

10/17/19 9:10 AM - 10:52 AM

There is a trickle of students in and out
of the library this morning and I join them at
the long tables to spy on my banner while it
went to work. Most people notice the banner,
some smile. Some stay with their heads in their
phones. I would say there is an average of 5
people per minute walking through the doors.
This proceeds for 2 hours.

At around 10:50 AM, two library employees
walk in. The one in the red vest exclaims
"What the fork is this?" — Obviously flabber-
gasted, possibly angry. She proceeds to take
a photo and at this point I can't tell if its out
of amusement or if she's going to turn it in to
campus security.

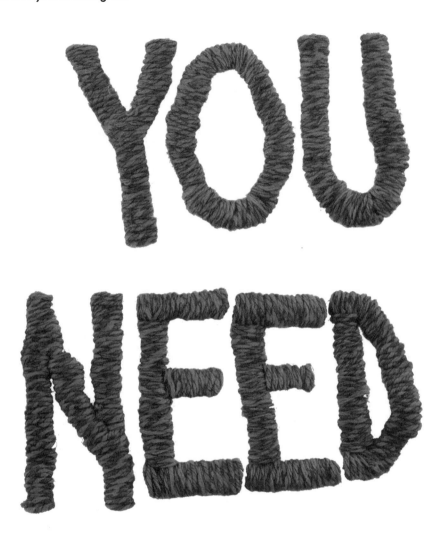

She smiles at the other employee standing next to her. The other employee is wearing a black vest. Black vest says something like "oh but it's harmless..."
"But we still can't have it!" red vest says stormily and marches out in disbelief that someone, somewhere has introduced a bump in the road of a usual Thursday morning.

I don't go up to them to talk about the banner, afraid they'd cuff me right then and there; is it the truism that cuts or the passive intervention of placing the banner in the library? Do they feel violated as recipients of unsolicited advice? Dumbfounded by the absurdity of an intervention in a library; a place as neutral as Switzerland? As soon as the vested ladies turn around I slink over and take the banner down. I remain incognito and sit back at the long work tables to observe what ensues.

Four new library employees enter staggeringly to scan the area. Some seem angry, some bewildered, some confused; all of the library employees look like children on an Easter egg hunt. Did I just make them have a good time?

I do not feel suddenly struck by the epiphany that I should stop reading. I do not even believe my banner. It was like reading the words "you can't read." This seems to be a classic case of overcompensation: it is childish of me to think that the answer is to stop reading altogether.

However, I like planting a surprise for the staff and that wasn't reading. I like to think my banner seasoned an otherwise bland day for the librarians, suddenly distinguishable from the rest. While trying to figure out what I can consume less of in my life, it seems I've found that I need something else: disruption.

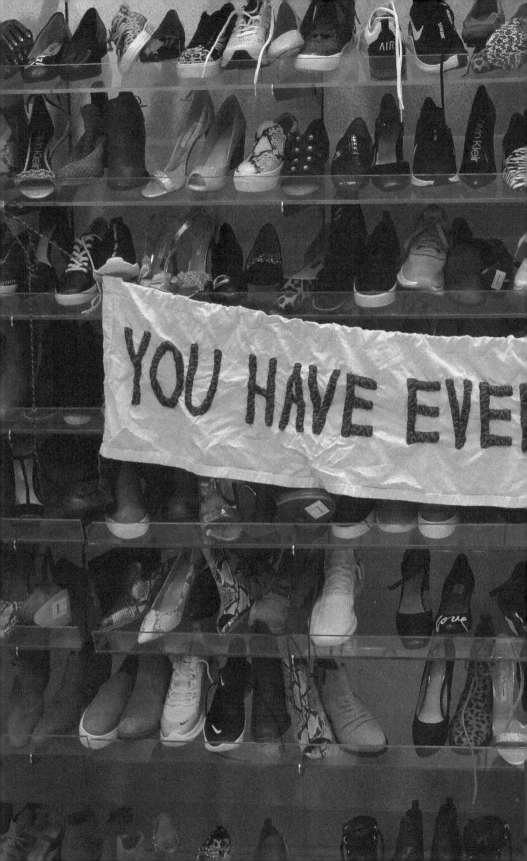

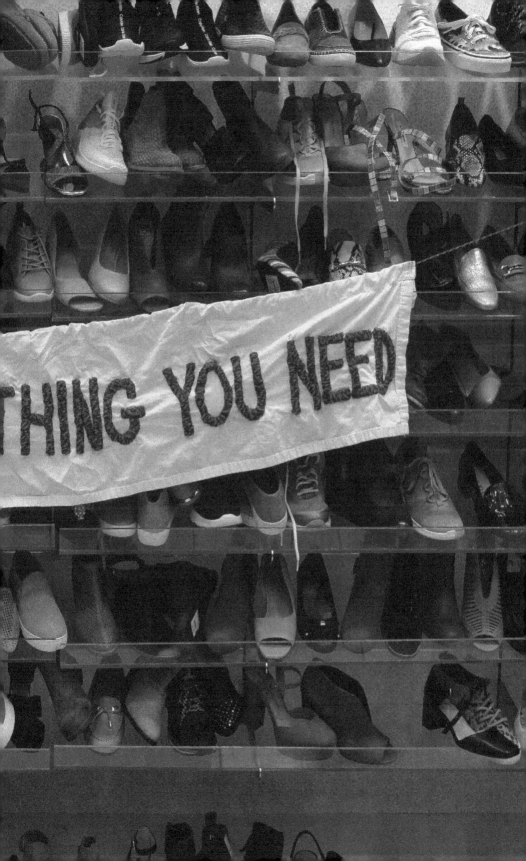

## After my run at the library, I want

to find a place with both elements of disruption and truth. I land on the Briarwood Mall: home of department stores and kiosks, frozen yogurt and strong perfume.

I venture to the Briarwood Mall with very low expectations for tolerance of my project. This is brick and mortar materialism, no conspicuous, targeted Instagram advertisement, no proceeds are going to a charitable cause: we are in the business of buying for pleasure. While physical commerce spaces are increasingly transitioning to online platforms, becoming more ubiquitous, more ingrained into our daily lives, I admire the clarity of intentions at the mall whether I fundamentally agree with them or not. The honesty almost holds me back. But then I see a pair of hideous high heels designed to look like a suit and tie and muster on. Someone needs me to tell them they don't need these shoes and all adjacent horrors.

What are you Looking at?

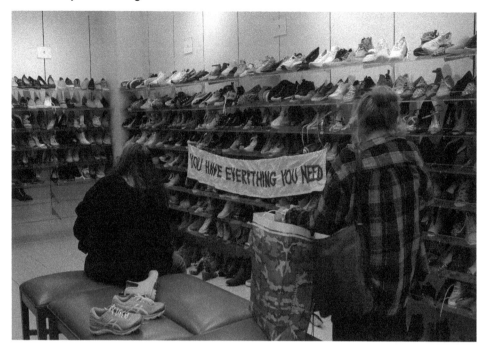

10/30/19 2:57 PM - 4:01 PM

I feel like an outsider, unaffected by the merchandise cluttering my vision: has the burden of consumption been lifted from my shoulders — am I godsend, salvation in girl form, or do I just not like anything here? With the banner in my hands, I feel protected, like I have a mission of the higher order to accomplish.

I pace Von Maur, the most luxurious store in the mall. Past the pyramid of fall booties, I hit the clearance shoe room, out of employee sight. Shoppers come and go, some sit to contemplate shoes and I see them gaze at the banner. No one asks about the banner, but no one buys shoes. Victory? I move on.

I approach the make-up counter at Von Maur and ask if I can hang it around the cosmetics for a photo. I explain that I am an art student with a project in which I photograph a banner in different contexts. She calls her manager. After the call fails to go through, she says "you know what that means for us…You know that's against what we are going for…" I say I understand the implications. She says "so what are you going to do with an art degree after college?"

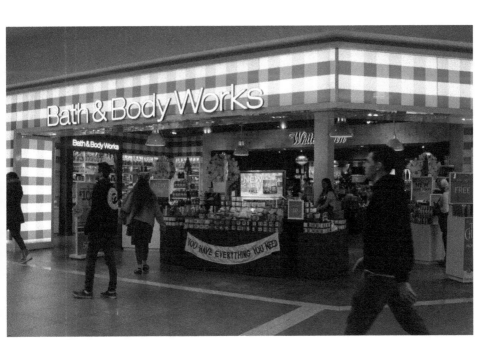

Never mind that most shoppers who pass by are clutching their bags like buoys post-capsized at sea, eyes starry from the glass window displays; the slight abhorrence of store policy thrills me. I am having capital-F fun. I slink around from Bath and Body Works to H&M, to the Pagoda jewelry stand in the center of the mall. While everyone around me is occupied by getting what they need, I too, in my own sense, am occupied by the same thing.

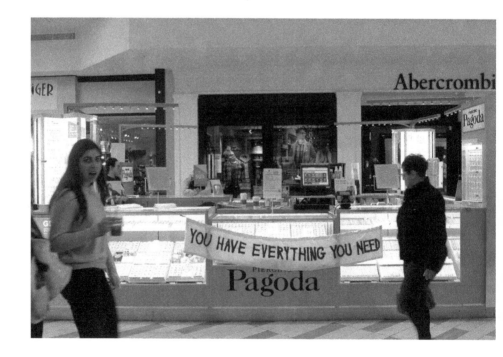

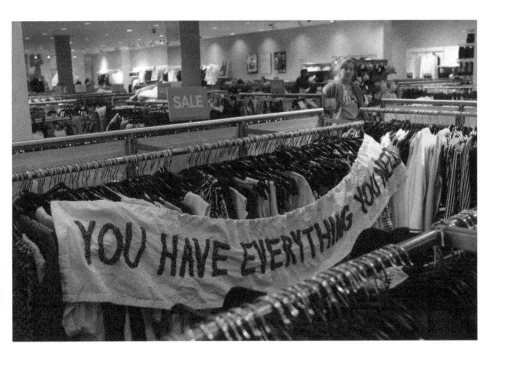

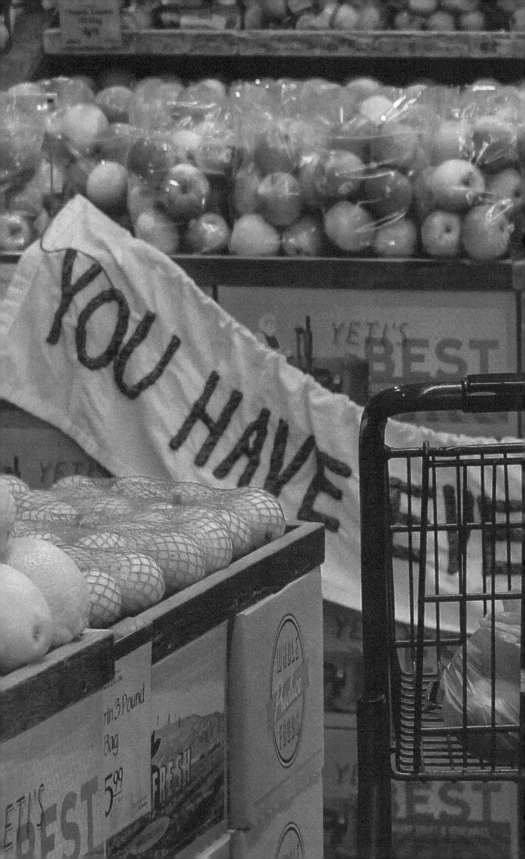

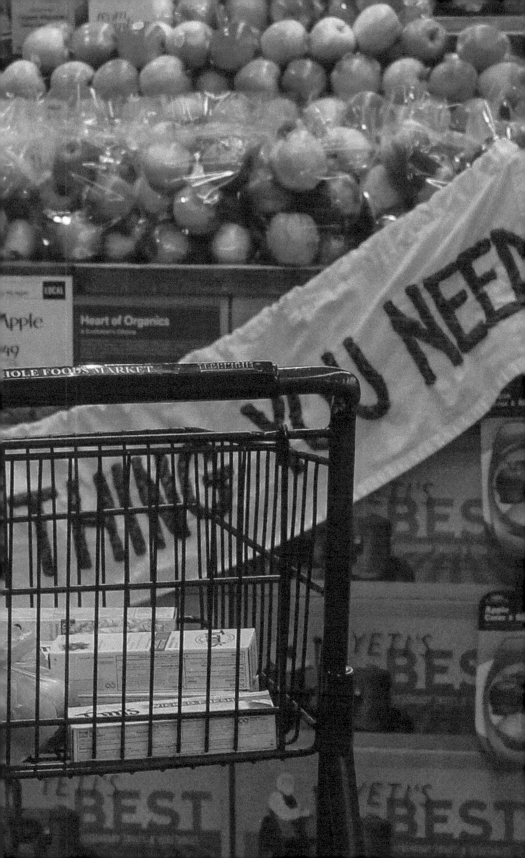

**I am accompanying my sister Paige** on a mid-afternoon trip to Whole Foods. This store contains a similar volume of goods as the stores in the mall and while food is essential, Whole Foods is known for being luxuriously extra. Will my banner hold up in this context?

We enter at the produce section; I scan for a wide surface to display the banner. After a few lumpy tries on top of squash, I hang the banner from a display of apples. I pace nearby, recover from the adrenaline, and check out the lettuce. It's 2:51 PM.

The pace of Whole Foods is leisurely: 5-10 people shop in the produce area at a time. I hear a few snickering at the sign. One man laughs, makes eye contact with me, then starts singing a happy tune to his wife who affectionately shushes him. I peek into their cart: apples, eggs, sliced ham, and coffee beans. It looks methodical. I don't see the signs of rampant consumerism. I stalk my sister who is buying sliced cheese. The view from the deli is perfect.

It's 3:03 PM and this feels like endurance art — a Sisyphean climb in front of an audience — however, no one else seems to see the mountain. Or maybe they see the mountain as a ski mogul. Three Whole Foods employees pass by and I think they are IN ON IT: one of the employees, I later learn is named Bailey, acknowledges me with a smile as she unloads produce. Another employee, Brian, gives me a wink, although I'm not certain he saw the sign. These exchanges seem like an unspoken pact that I am on their side: it's us against the indulgent clientele.

At 3:17 PM I dive into the cosmetics aisle
to watch perplexed apple-buyers. A lady with
stunning auburn hair parks her cart in front
of the apples and takes a few steps back. Her
feet are in fifth position as she bows to read the
banner. Her head swivels and then returns to
her shopping list.

I come out of the aisle smelling like an
Aunt's hug during the holidays (I've tested
every cream blush). It is 3:37 PM and I notice
the banner has been removed after I briefly
looked away. I look around for an employee
and scurry over to the customer service desk.
The three employees have not heard of my
banner; we track down Bailey. This is the part
where I learn her name.

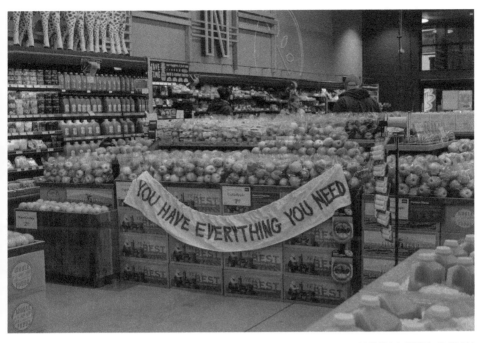

11/1/19 2:57 PM - 3:37 PM

**EW:** Hi, my name is Erin. I'm working on a project where I photograph a banner in public places. Have you seen my banner here today?

**Bailey:** Yes, I did see it! It is so cute. I don't know where it went. I didn't take it down. I saw it while I was working.

After a brief chase, Bailey finds the banner in the break room. Mike from the deli counter grabbed it. When I ask Bailey if he said anything, she responds: "I have no idea what goes through that man's head most of the time."

What I'm learning is that the banner will always get taken down. The answer isn't because it offends shoppers' sensibilities, it's due to store policy. Passersby will largely ignore the banner. This project is suddenly excruciatingly predictable. I'm starting to feel dumb.

Also, it might be true that people need things. People need apples. People need new shoes when they've worn through the toes and broken the zipper. People need their weekly round up of eggs, coffee beans, ham, and apples. Through my spastic sign placing I've decided that I have the authority to dictate what people can and can't have. I'm seeking a place that does not insult or confront; can this sign be harmonious with its surroundings?

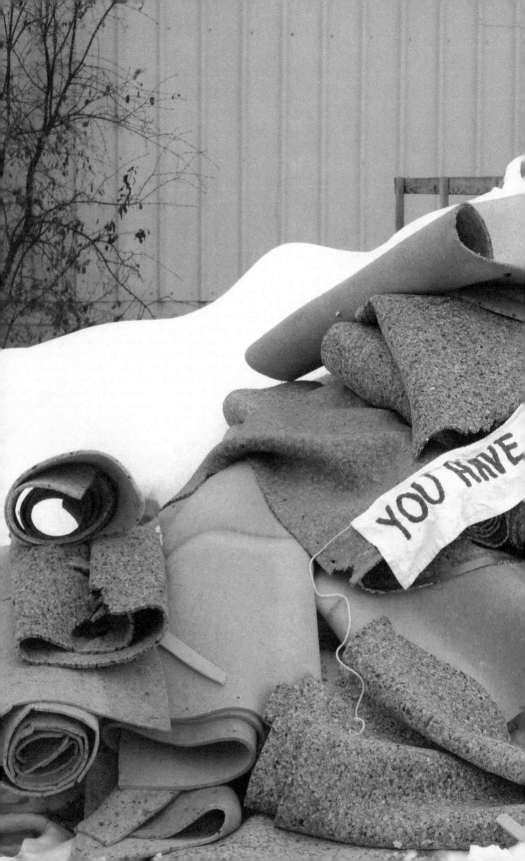

...THING YOU NEED

11/15/19 3:56 PM

## My favorite craft store moved locations.

I learn this the hard way: a closed sign post-
ed on the cloudy window of the old location.
Dumbfounded with my friend Madalyn, I
U-turn on the dead-end street; our car was
pulsing to the beat of the song "Kick it to Me"
by Sammy Rae. Driving leisurely, chin cocked,
lyrics spilling out of my mouth, my eye catches
a pile of junk. Trash! In the dumpster! Luckily,
I have the banner and camera in the back of
my car for a moment like this.

   This seems to be the obvious answer to my
qualms found at the grocery store: the banner
is not out of place nor in a place. No one can
take it down because the dumpster simulta-
neously belongs to no one and everyone. The
difference between trash and everything else
is that someone decided no one should want or
need this ever again. The banner agrees with
its setting.

I make fresh tracks in the shallow snow,
running out to get a wider angle. The mountain
of rolled carpets and insulation looks as deli-
cate as a pile of satin ribbons. They are beautiful. Interrupting the awe, I feel a devil tapping
my shoulder. The banner is out of place.

I labeled something beautiful as something
undesirable. Whatever I place the banner
on, my mark is authoritative. The banner is
just as confrontational as it was in places of
commerce: I decide where the line is drawn
between abundance and absence. Someone
decided these materials go to the dump, but
they aren't
worthless. I feel despondent— the one place I
thought would be an easy yes is also complicat-
ed. I retrieve the banner and hustle back to the
car.
"Got the shot?" Madalyn asked.
"Yeah..." I say like a deflating balloon.

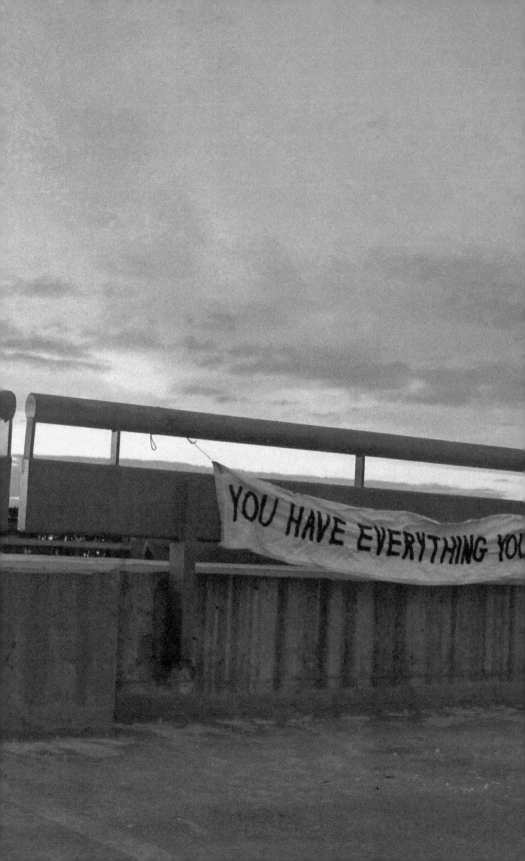

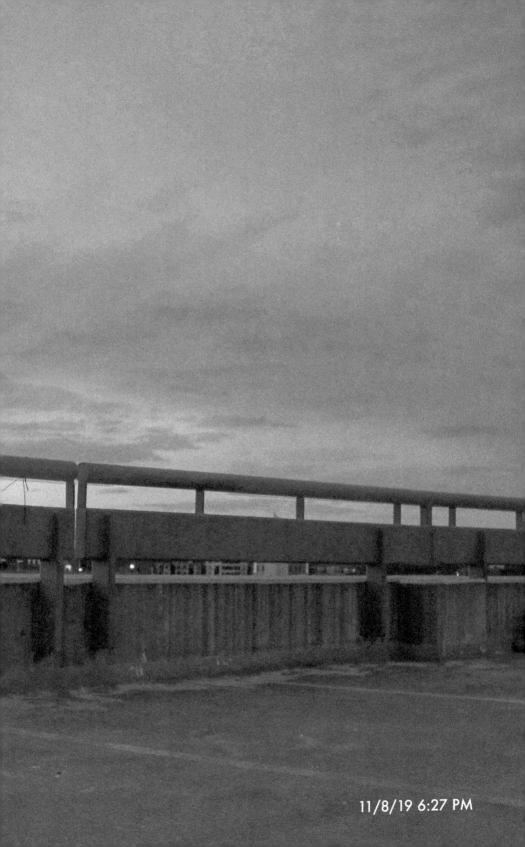
11/8/19 6:27 PM

# I had an idea for a performance

piece earlier this year that involved dressing
in business attire and cinematically sprinting
downtown as if I'm late to work — work being
watching the sunrise from a parking structure.
The piece has obvious holes: sleepy Ann Arbor
does not have a vibrant walk-to-work culture,
nor is there a parking structure with a clear
eastern view.

Friday evening I woke up from a cat nap to
a sky made of brilliant pinks and purples. I rub
my blurry eyes. I operate on whim. I decide
I'm going to try to recover my banner from
project purgatory.

I sprint out of the house and bike to
Thompson street like hell on wheels. The
urgency I felt transcended being late for class,
waiting tables at the French restaurant, the
moment I realize a first date is not going well.
Time abides by nature only and if I miss the
setting sun, it won't dip upwards for an encore.

I double-step seven flights of stairs to the
top of the parking structure and let out a sigh
of relief/exhaustion. The gray, empty structure
floor reflects the sky, turning into a lilac blue.
I am between the two color palettes — the
expanse seems infinite as I'm above the street
noise and the skyline. The banner looks different set against the sky. I squint my eyes and
imagine it flying on the tail of an airplane: free,
unsolicited advice in the most free, unsolicited space I know. It seems to me I am exactly
where I need to be.

# What are you Looking at?

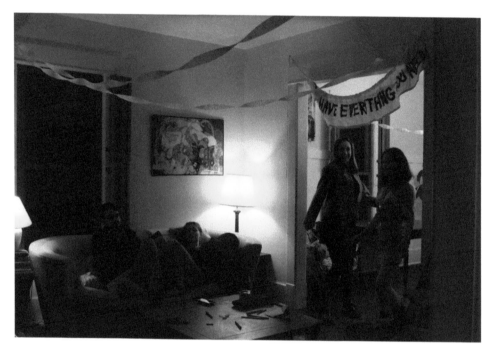

10/25/19 9:32 PM

## Through all of this I remembered

my roommates Katie and Madalyn put the banner up during Madalyn's birthday party. We loved the phrase and they love me for my work even when it's bad. I look at this authentic capture — a celebratory buzz hummed throughout the air, our ceilings trapezed with decorations, friends giddy or resting in anticipation of an energetic night. The night went onward, we drank wine and danced. The banner remained in the background as our touchstone.

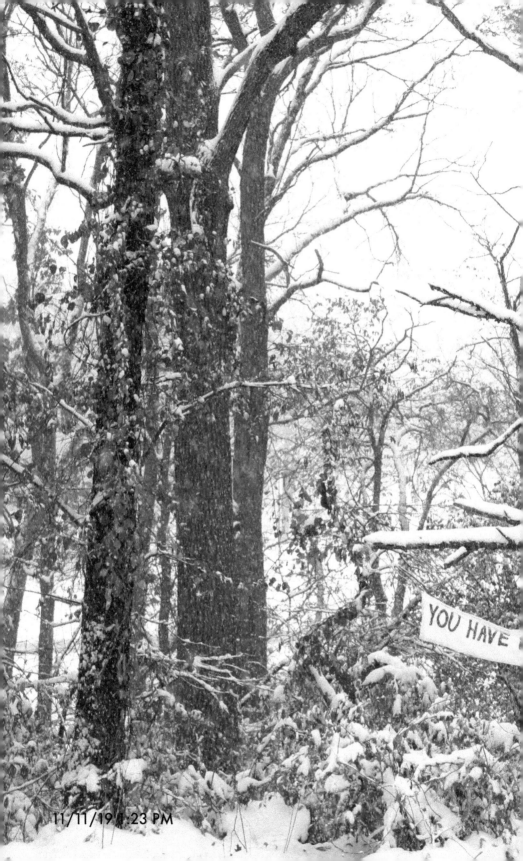

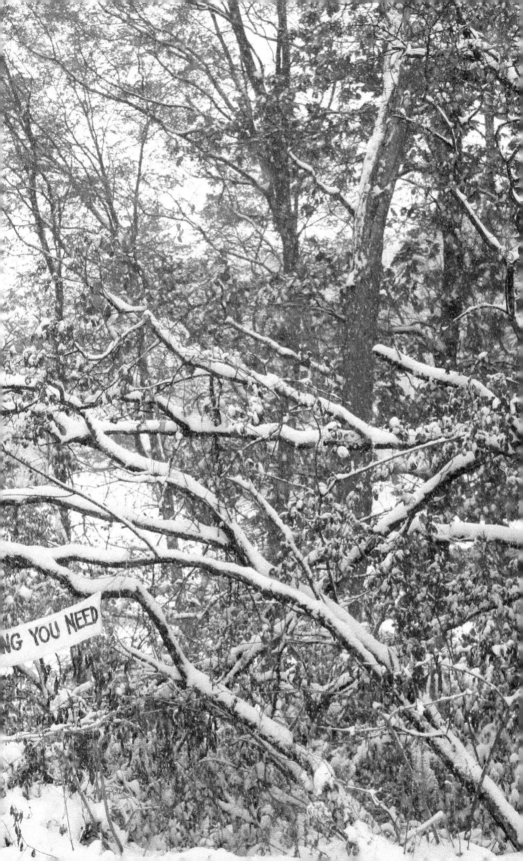

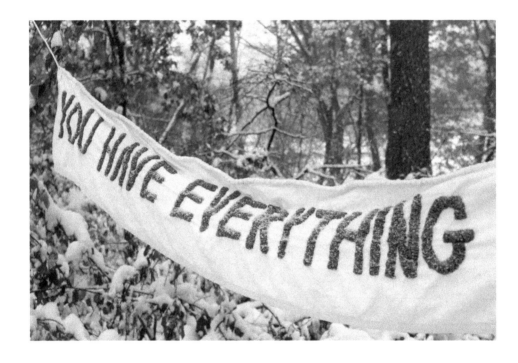

## This is the first snow of the season.

It came down overnight as thick as the frosting on a sheet cake. My bones still seem to carry the sun, so I ran out the door this morning without a heavy coat and stomped around fearlessly. During a break in my day, I went outside to the woods by my school to admire the blinding whites.

The banner feels celebratory, harmonious, and accepted by the branches. I imagine that the banner sprouted from the tree limbs and dropped the way flags unroll from castle windows during celebrations, trumpets play in the background with confetti sprinkling the sky. This feels like a finish line.

When I finish this essay, close this book, eat this apple, do I actually have everything I need? Could you lock me in a vault and not come back for a few days? Humans are very needy. We need to be fed and watered daily. We need love and affection, vitamin D, and material things. Ironically, this project became a litmus test for what we need. But I still question: how can we have everything we need and be aware that we don't need everything?

What I've figured out is that giving unsolicited advice makes me feel bad. And sometimes,
I love to be a spectacle. Maybe this project
was really all to service my needs. I loved
seeing the whistling man in the grocery store
and I loved having a sassy conversation with
the makeup clerk. I loved chasing the sunset
and dancing with friends under the banner.
Perhaps what we truly need is something to
bring a jolt of joy, and for some people shoes
shaped into tuxedos do it for them. Sometimes
those joys can be buying unnecessary shoes,
but if we fill our days with more living from the
square foot in which we are standing (dancing,
talking, running...), we might realize we feel
full after all. ■

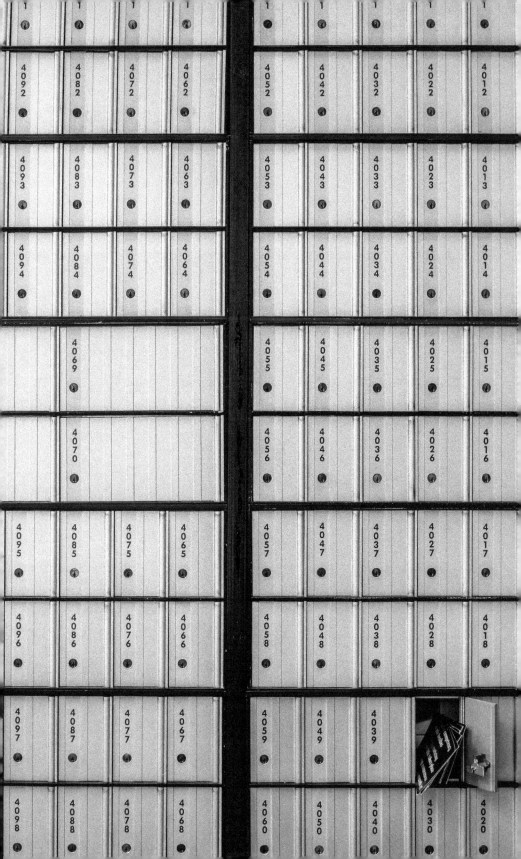

**What is competency in life besides**

**1. Deeply noticing where life takes place**

**2. A loving awareness and interaction with it?**

# What have you noticed lately?

**Erin Wakeland**
PO Box 4029
Ann Arbor, MI
48106-4029

Hello! I'm happy to have found you. Once you respond to the above prompt, drop this postcard into the mail to participate in project, *What are you Looking at?*. Learn more at erinraywakeland.com. All best, Erin Wakeland

**This winter, I placed 100 postcards**
with this message— stamped and addressed
to my P.O. box— for strangers to discover.
Partially looking for confirmation that I can
believe this manifesto and partially probing
for a connection with city-dwellers that closely
examine newspaper racks on their walk home.

I'm curious how people would live if they
believed competency in life was simply being
attentive. Instead of accomplishments and ac-
colades measuring success, what if it was about
how well we notice the world? Every smile as
you wave pedestrians on from your car grants
you a gold star on your life-success chart. We'd
go for more streetlight-lit walks in the dead
of winter. Maybe we'd host roadkill funerals
and spend afternoons following ants until they
duck into their sand hills.

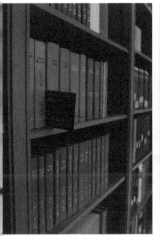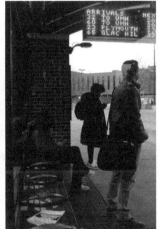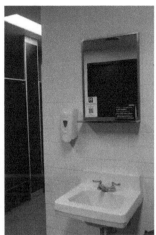

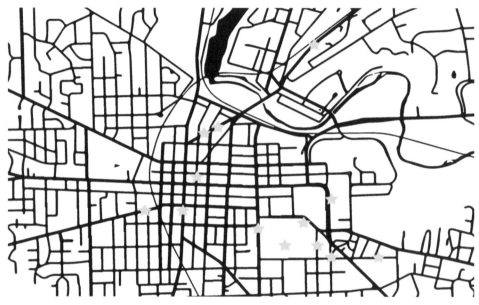

Postcard placements in Ann Arbor, MI.

I loved placing the postcards about town: I milled about the library to wedge them between tight shelves of orange books and float one over an atlas splayed open on Michigan. One became a mouse pad in the computer lab and I dropped another on the library's marble steps to look as if it precariously fell out of my hand. I stuck a few on giant rocks across the Diag with a tiny rock to weigh them down. I left them on bus stop benches, telephone polls, newspaper racks, and bathroom sinks. I left a few at the bookstore, my favorite coffee shop, and later, Madalyn paraded me around her workplace, the Farmers Market, to scatter them between farmers and produce and pastries.

The first time I checked my P.O. box was two weeks after I first placed them. During the two weeks I went away for Thanksgiving break, I felt uncomfortably pulled from this spider web I'd strung across the city.

My boyfriend Julian met me outside the post office. My walk took longer than usual because I was dragging my feet in anticipation. I couldn't preview the results. Asking strangers to do things for your art project isn't always successful, especially when it involves more than one step (filling out the prompt then placing it in the mail instead of your desk drawer for 3 months). I know that I would let the postcard mingle with my papers and become acquainted with the insides of my books, turning it into a bookmark with the intention that now it's with me all the time so when I feel inspired to write, I will. But I won't. I'd grow attached and never part with it. I come to my P.O. box with this knowledge.

I slide the key in easily. Honestly I'd wished for a little more trouble to stall the reveal. But the box pops open, hollow without postcards. Julian and I let out a groan.
"I'm not disappointed that there weren't any, but I'm disappointed that I was correct to assume I wouldn't get any back," I say to Julian. I promise to him that I won't check it again for a few weeks.

The next time I checked, I went by myself. I crouch down to where my P.O. box is the height of my shin and wiggle the key in.

I open to see one prized postcard.

# What have you noticed lately?

A wedge of a sliced Halloween pumpkin has been left to rot at the base of a tree near my house. But instead of rotting, it froze! The exposed edges of the slice looks like rock crystals. certainly not so It's hard to imagine anyone cutting through this. the stringy things that get all over your hands when you carve one are frozen white, like a dense spider web criss-crossing the bowl of the pumpkin slice.

**Erin Wakeland**
PO Box 4029
Ann Arbor
48106-4029

A few weeks later I receive 3 more.

## What have you noticed lately?

It's important to seek
new knowledge,
reflect on the end
how it applies to
self. It goes beyond
our own awareness
and expands our
possibility of growth.

08 DEC 2015 PM 15 L

**Erin Wakeland**
PO Box 4029
Ann Arbor, MI
48106-4029

Hello! I'm happy to have found you. Once you respond to the above prompt, drop this postcard into the mail to participate in a project, *What are you looking at?* Learn more at erinraywakeland.com. All best, Erin Wakeland

## What have you noticed lately?

I walk a lot to clear my head. I especially like strolling through the graveyard across from Stockwell (Forest Hill Cemetery). Plots in older zones tend to have a large family marker and smaller individual stones. (Once I noticed a stone with my last name and discovered relatives from 100 years ago that my grandparents were even unaware of.)

A family stone deep in the cemetery caught my eye with the last name Butts (ha, ha), but it presented a mystery: It has 4 names and lifespans, but a William Henry Butts was missing his death year. That itself is not uncommon (it's cheaper to engrave most of the stone before it's installed and update it after death). William was born in 1857, though, so he should be dead by now. I looked it up on my phone right there. William, turns out, was a professor of mathematics at the university. He's buried with his parents, who died in 1875 and 1906, and his wife, who died in 1935. He died in 1941. His death date is missing because he was the last one to die.

I emailed the cemetery to ask if they would add a date, but they didn't understand my request, and wouldn't do anything for free or without the family's permission anyway. I've thought about adding his death year myself with chalk or paint. I wonder if anyone would notice or care. The crows roost in that cemetery during the day before they float at sunset and roost around the diag and law quad at night. I wonder if Professor Butts would have liked this or found it annoying.

    —Leila Mullison
    lrmull@umich.edu

**Erin Wakeland**
PO Box 4029
Ann Arbor, MI
48106-4029

Hello! I'm happy to have found you. Once you respond to the above prompt, drop this postcard into the mail to participate in project, *What are you Looking at?* Learn more at erinraywakeland.com. All best, Erin Wakeland

# What have you noticed lately?

Trees - sprawling *bare* branches
majestic crowns opening up to
the sky, looking so different
in the fall, near winter grounds.
    Behavior + feelings about transition
about change, about $, about
jobs + careers and about the two
sides to every person + me! ☮

Hello! I'm happy to have found you. Once you respond to
the above prompt, drop this postcard into the mail to
participate in project, *What are you looking at?* Learn
more at erinraywakeland.com. All best, Erin Wakeland

**Erin Wakeland**
PO Box 4029
Ann Arbor, MI
48106-4029

And on my third check, I find 9 more.

## What have you noticed lately?

"Who is it that sees through
these eyes
hears through these ears?"

Thank You for this
this Loving Awareness

Erin Wakeland
PO Box 4029
Ann Arbor, MI
48106-4029

Hello! I'm happy to have found you. Once you respond to
the above prompt, drop this postcard into the mail to
participate in project, *What are you Looking at?* Learn
more at erinraywakeland.com. All best, Erin Wakeland

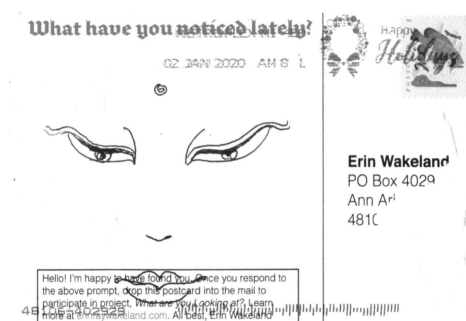

**What have you noticed lately!**

02 JAN 2020   AM 6  L

**Erin Wakeland**
PO Box 4029
Ann Ar'
481C

Hello! I'm happy to have found you. Once you respond to the above prompt, drop this postcard into the mail to participate in project, *What are you Looking at?* Learn more at erinraywakeland.com. All best, Erin Wakeland

**What have you noticed lately?**

METROPLEX MI 480

02 JAN 2020    AM 7  L

Rain drops

on pine needles —

the sky in
    their droop

**Erin Wakeland**
PO Box 4029
Ann Arbor, MI
48106-4029

Hello! I'm happy to have found you. Once you respond to
the above prompt, drop this postcard into the mail to
participate in project, *What are you Looking at?* Learn
more at erinraywakeland.com. All best, Erin Wakeland

**What have you noticed lately?**

12/15/19 AZ MI

People are lonely. They
don't ~~simple~~ smile as
much, ~~then don't know you~~ if they don't know you. Sadly I think

They long for human
interaction but there
is A shyness which
is growing. We need to open
up and LIVE life to th~

Awesome
idea

Jollest. Roast JOHN

Roos Roast Coffee!

Great Project!

**Erin Wakeland**
PO Box 4029
Ann Arbor, MI
48106-4029

Hello! I'm happy to have found you. Once you respond to the above prompt, drop this postcard into the mail to participate in project, *What are you Looking at?* Learn more at erinraywakeland.com. All best, Erin Wakeland

## What have you noticed lately?

The bigger, older oak trees seem to be suffering. I hope I am noticing this because I stare at the same big trees in town all the time, and that ones I don't stare at/notice are doing fine. . . . Nick Durrie

**Erin Wakeland**
PO Box 402ɛ
Ann Arbor, MI
48106-4029

Hello! I'm happy to have found you. Once you respond to the above prompt, drop this postcard into the mail to participate in project, *What are you looking at?* Learn more at erinraywakeland.com. All best, Erin Wakeland

**What have you noticed lately?**

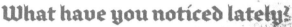

I have noticed
That it is getting
darker earlier.

**Erin Wakeland**
PO Box 4029
Ann Arbor, MI
48106-4

Hello! I'm happy to have found you. Once you respond to
the above prompt, drop this postcard into the mail to
participate in project, *What are you Looking at?*. Learn
more at erinwaywakeland.com. All best, Erin Wakeland

# What have you noticed lately?

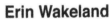

That it's not so
clear who, what,
I am.

**Erin Wakeland**
PO Box 4029
Ann Arbor, MI
48106-4029

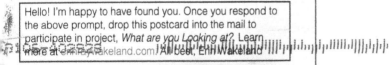

Hello! I'm happy to have found you. Once you respond to
the above prompt, drop this postcard into the mail to
participate in project, *What are you Looking at?* Learn
more at erinwakeland.com. All best, Erin Wakeland

## What have you noticed lately?

I've noticed that walking outside in the early morning light, with a little frost on the ground, is quite magical.

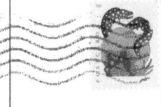

**Erin Wakeland**
PO Box 4029
Ann Arbor, '
4810C 4C

Hello! I'm happy to have found you. Once you respond to the above prompt, drop this postcard into the mail to participate in project, *What are you Looking at?*. Learn more at erinwakeland.com. All best, Erin Wakeland

## What have you noticed lately?

I just finished a deep conversation
with one of my friends. I notice
the tears leaving trails from where
they streaked down my face. I
notice a feeling of calmness after
unaddressed tension dissipates.
I love this project!
from Maine, with love,
Nico

Hello! I'm happy to have found you. Once you respond to
the above prompt, drop this postcard into the mail to
participate in project, *What are you Looking at?* Learn
more at erinfaywakeland.com. All best, Erin Wakeland

**Erin Wakeland**
PO Box 4029
Ann Arbor, MI
48106-4029

A month went by and I swing through the post office the way you check if you've turned off all the lights before leaving the house. Nothing. I chalk my total up to 13 postcards.

I keep them in my coat pocket to look at on bus rides. They are held together by the rubber band that came with last week's broccoli bunch. I interchange them like trading cards. A different one faces up each time so that I can be surprised for a split second. I do think about the other 87 postcards roaming this earth. Some might be in the recycling bin, or behind the counter of the bookstore. Some might have found their way onto a dorm room's wall or office desk. Maybe some people needed this reminder for longer than a writing prompt. But if a few people felt eager enough to share their thoughts with me, I feel content clutching onto these 13 postcards like group therapy. ∎

I'd like to hear from you too.
What have you noticed lately?

Email *erinwakeland@gmail.com* for a chat.

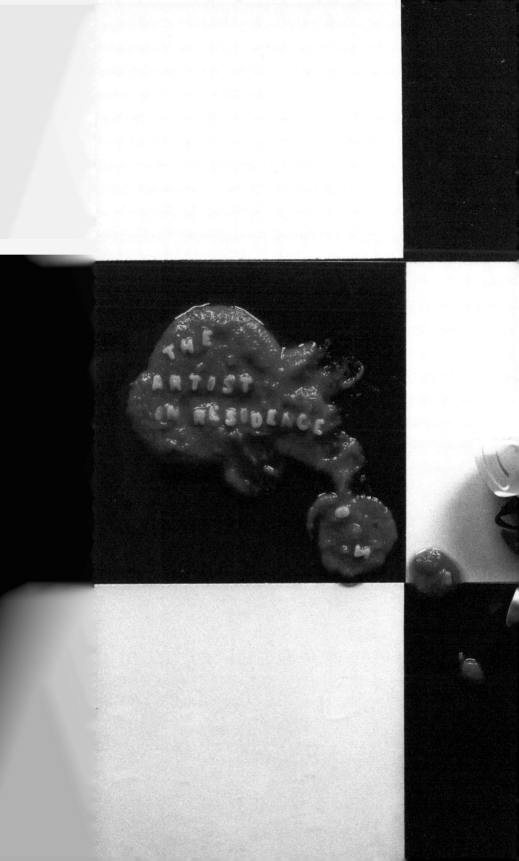

# What are you Looking at?

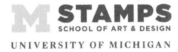

UNIVERSITY OF MICHIGAN

Hena Patel
Manager
Meijer Store
5645 Jackson Rd
Ann Arbor, MI 48103

Dear Hena Patel,

I am writing to propose myself as a Visiting Artist-in-Residence for the Meijer Superstore on Jackson Rd from November 11th to November 22th 2019.

Over the past thirty years, institutions not normally associated with art have welcomed artists into their doors. The Mall of America in Minnesota invites a single writer to spend five days writing poetry inspired by shoppers' experiences. Artists have taken up residence on moving Amtrak trains and at the Dollar Shave Club. The San Francisco Transfer and Recycling Center, a forty-seven-acre garbage dump, offers access to discarded materials to a small group of sculptors who work with found objects.

Over the next semester I, as an art major in the Stamps School of Art & Design at the University of Michigan, will be taking up residence at stores throughout Ann Arbor. My work as resident will involve observation, as my medium and subject is landscape painting and I will paint inspired by these contexts.

Retail stores, like Meijer, offer an encyclopedia array of ideas about packaging, presentation, and human interaction, and I would be excited to be a resident. I'll provide my own resources as I am not asking for any financial support from Meijer.

Creative work is essential to the intellectual and spiritual well-being of our culture. I appreciate your advocacy for the arts and would love to work as an artist-in-residence at Meijer.

You can reach me at erinray@umich.edu or (517)348-8195.

Stamps Professor Stephanie Rowden is overseeing the Artist-in-Residence project. She would be happy to provide a reference or further information. You can reach her at srowden@umich.edu.

All the best,

Erin Wakeland, BFA 2020

Adapted from a template created by Rebekah Modrak.

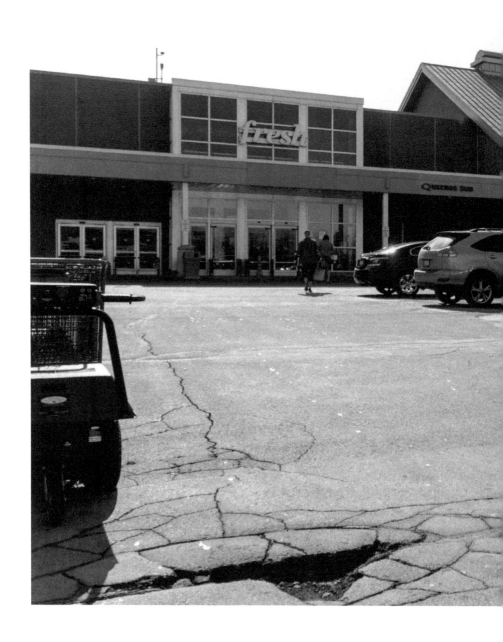

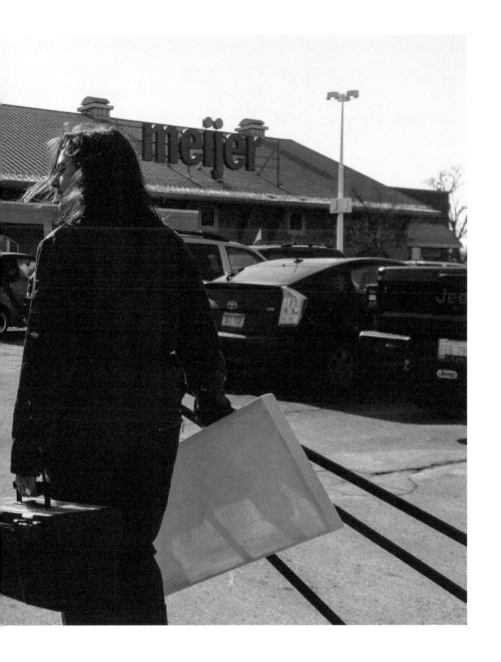

### Feb 10 1-3:30PM, Aisle 1

**I walk into Meijer as an artist-in-residence.**
The door greeter waves at me like any other
customer, but I dodge a conversation, worried
about getting flagged for mischief. I am an
artist-in-residence at Meijer. I remind myself
of this. Easel in hand, the blowing fans meant
to dry the welcome carpets instead glamorize
my entrance. I'm in uniform: my green cotton
jumpsuit holds paint on the surface and my
brushes in the front pockets. By painting in the
tradition of en plein air painters in the Meijer
superstore, I want to show that ordinary places
are filled with just as much mystique and beauty as Monet's garden; the French country-side;
dappled light at the water's edge.

I've been entertained by the grocery store
since childhood. I was always the first to help
my mom in exchange for a long look at the
packages and produce displays. I've always
thought this place was beautiful but I know
it's a chore for others. I wanted to display my
marvel in a way that prompts others to see it as
a visual playground.

As I walk through looking for a place to
set up, I notice the entire store is a new frontier
in which the ceiling perfectly crops my view
into an elongated horizontal landscape. Visions
like the colorful produce aisles and uni-color
cracker displays make for a visual feast. I decide to choose my painting locations arbitrarily,
but aisle one seems like a good place to start.
The pickle aisle.

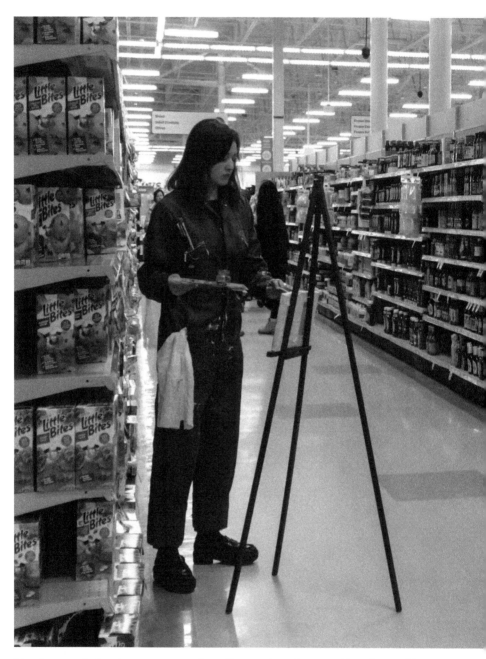

I begin my painting three rows up, where Famous Dave's meets Mt. Olive pickles.

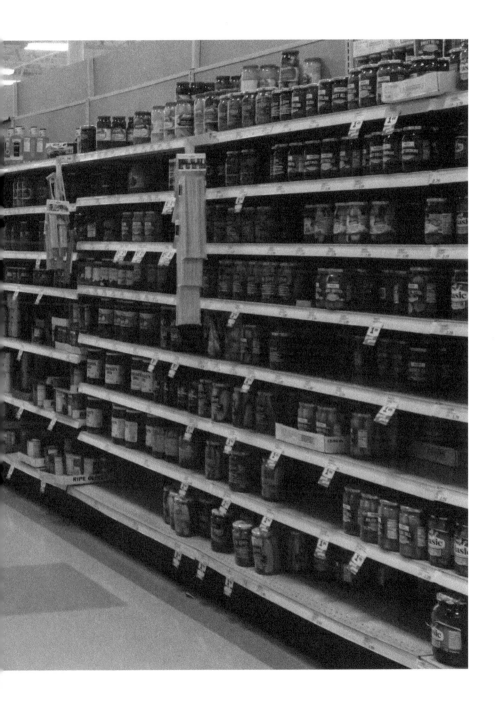

Cindy from the Deli counter is the first to approach me as I set up. She is small, smiling, and wearing a hat that has an embroidered block of cheese on the front.

"What are you doing here? Painting?" She says warmly. I am quick to sputter my status as Hena Patel's artist-in-residence, but it slides off her back. Cindy was just curious. While the word of my residency may not have traveled at all, no one here is looking to trouble me. They might not understand what I'm doing, but I'm out of the bounds of Meijer mischief. How do employees handle this strange behavior? They smile, nod, and ask a few questions.

Shoppers pass by and I am impressed by their confidence. They approach me to give out words of encouragement and peek behind my shoulder. Shoppers pause for a few minutes at most to watch me looking deeply at the fermented foods.

COMMON QUESTIONS:
why are you doing this?
who are you doing this for?
Is this for the store?
Did the store hire you?
Do you work for Meijer?
Is this for class?
Is this for you or meijer?
where will these be shown?
Why this spot?
(when not flowers) Why not flowers?
(when not fruit) Why not fruit?
Will you get me in the shot?
Where are the cookies?
Can you point me to the _____?

COMMON EXCLAMATIONS:
I love to paint too.
I love that you are doing this.
I want to peek.
I just want to watch.
Very good.
Oh how great.
I loved art but it couldn't pay the bills.

I like to make people guess exactly what I'm looking at. The little game of eye spy usually does nothing for them. When I ask they often get the location wrong. And I blush, saying "Close! It's actually 5 rows down and on the other side of the shelf!" — Not close at all.

As I paint into the afternoon, employees joke with me as they restock the shelves, and another pair offers my next location to be aisle 8 where they are stationed. I feel very supported by the institution of Meijer, perhaps even coddled. I find myself nearing the end of my painting. I pack up, wave goodbye to my friends at the Deli, the door greeter, and then drive away.

What are you Looking at?

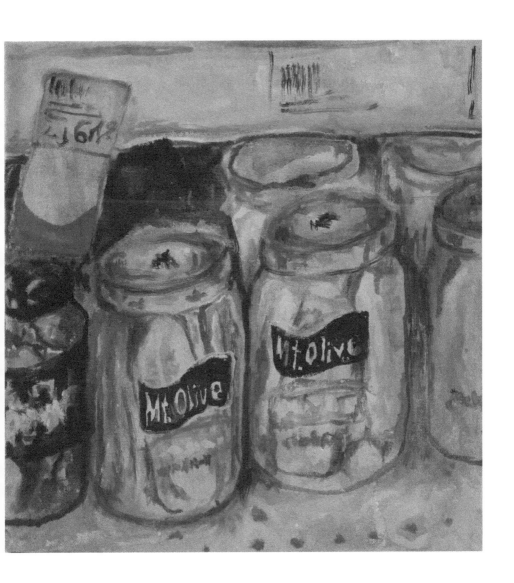

## Feb 15 12:30-4:00PM, Produce

I set up camp in a produce aisle, gazing at the avocados. I am drawn to the color variance amongst the avocados: dark brown, green, red, and purple hues lay against the lilac-colored cardboard. Immediately, I run into a customer that had spotted me last time. He joyfully asks me what I'm painting today. I make friends with the produce stocker, Aaron, whose hands scurry in and out of my frame. Time to work.

NEW QUESTIONS:
What is she doing, Mom?
Can I see?
Can I take your picture?
Why here?


NEW EXCLAMATIONS:
LOOK!
Gauguin! I mean Gogh! *Van*

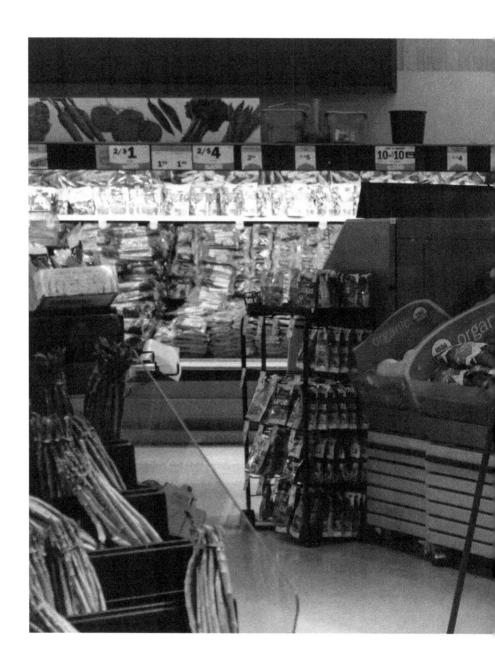

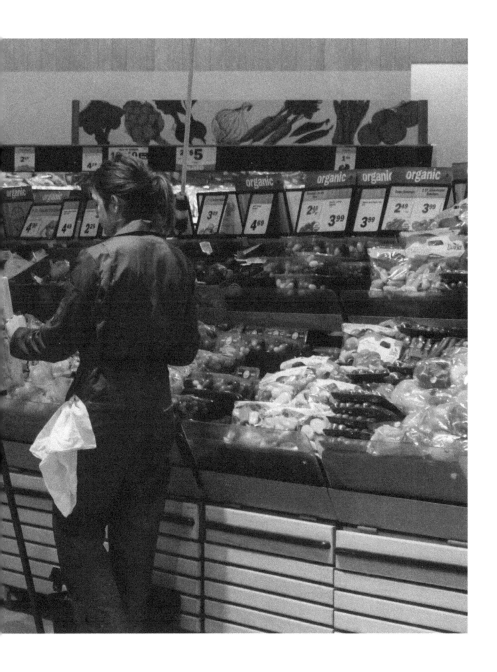

Kids accompany their parents on a Saturday afternoon grocery run. Even when their parents point me out, some kids aren't shocked by my presence. They say, "I do this at home too" or give me a look that says "lady, your painting doesn't look like avocados." On the occasion I'm met with wondrous eyes squatting between their mother's legs and the 24-pack of soda resting on the bottom shelf of the cart. I must be a bit magical to them.

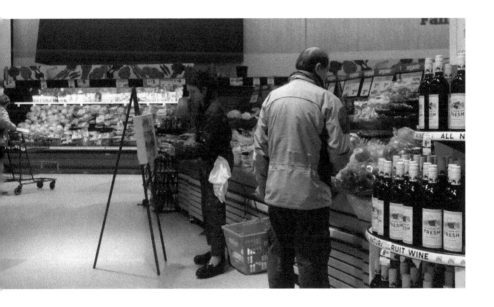

I find Meijer to be a bit magical in return. It's its own metropolis: this superstore appears to have its own local governance, golf cart transportation, and boroughs (food, clothing, equipment, etc.). Shoppers move fluently through the store and bring their cross-country finds with them. They aren't afraid to interact with me or annoyed that I disrupt the flow.

Later on in the day, an older man in a black
fleece zip up with a cap and glasses over his
glossy skin leans on his cart like a crutch and
says to me: "Most landscape paintings are
dreary with a dilapidated barn and gray sky.
And I think why not fix the plank and make it
sunny?"
I'm thinking he's on to me. Edging towards the
conversation I hope to have— one of expand-
ing which landscapes we deem beautiful and
attention-worthy— I ask him what he thinks
about this scene of avocados.
"I think it's fine. If it were any darker I
wouldn't like it but I'm no expert."
"You've got some paint on your chin" he ends
with and carts off.

I'm realizing that while my presence chang-
es the shopping experience for people, I am
perhaps the only one deeply aware of the mar-
velous differences in texture and color of the
avocados on cardboard; of the way pickle jars
retain hues of blue, green, and yellow; of the
modular shapes made with glimmering glass.

I'm enthralled because I've given this scene the attention necessary for fascination. While I chose my placements arbitrarily, I no longer see the aisles as one of many. I am seeing the store differently than when I first arrived, and sometimes I'm not seeing the store at all: I'm absorbed in the beauty of my subjects. This is something that is totally normal in nature, I beg why not in Meijer?

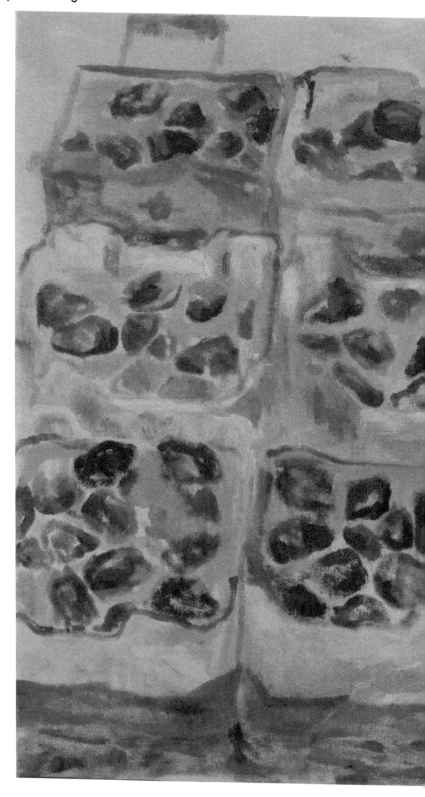

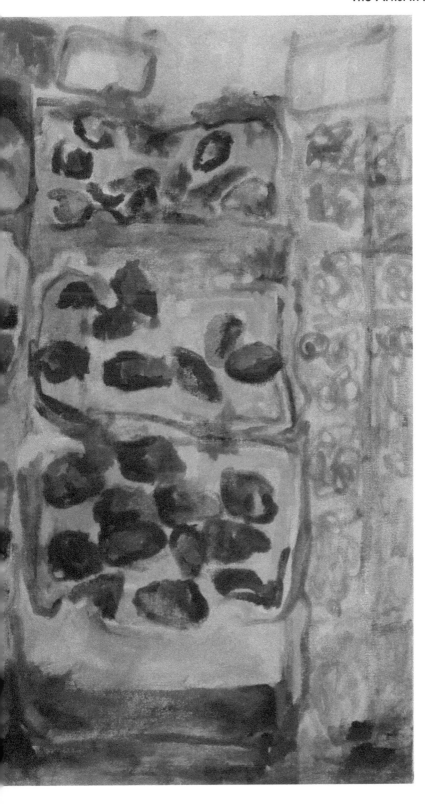

## Feb 16 1-3:30PM, Dairy

With a long, horizontal canvas in tow, I
stand in between cheese coolers for the best
landscape view of the dairy aisles. I get com-
fortable under the fluorescent lights. If Meijer
were its own metropolis, I'm on the shoulder
of a heavily trafficked road; the prime spot for
small talk, quick glances, and glares from afar.

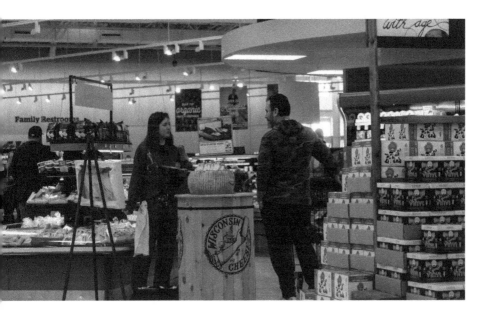

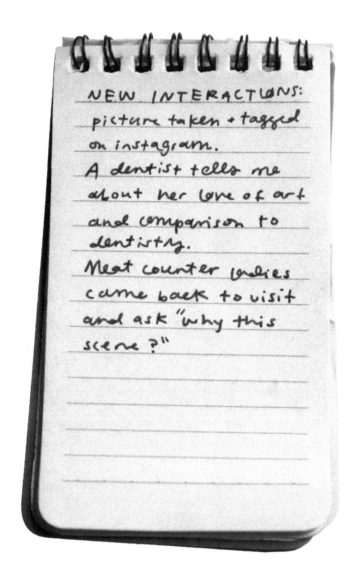

NEW INTERACTIONS:
picture taken + tagged
on instagram.
A dentist tells me
about her love of art
and comparison to
dentistry.
Meat counter ladies
came back to visit
and ask "why this
scene?"

A cheerful woman stops me and first said:
"Can I take your picture to show my students?
I'm a painter too!" I said yes and she promises
to text it to me. Her name is Miji.
"Usually you think of landscape paintings of
the outdoors but this is brilliant!"
Miji finds her husband and calls him over to
see my painting. Her husband is not as amused,
says "That's great honey!" and with a smile
slowly carts away toward the bananas.
     Miji said she understands how there are
so many crevices and interesting scenes to
paint here, that I must be wonderfully occupied. She's teaching her students observational
painting and asks me how I thought of
this project.

Miji understands my reference to en plein air painting, and was the only shopper to acknowledge it. But I like to think that while others might not have the term at the tip of their tongues, the argument that I was making was widely understood: the ordinary can be fascinating and it is a joyful discovery to come upon.

I'm finishing the landscape while realizing that I will miss this artist-in-residency. While I may not have made people see differently, I made the grocery store a new place for them in those moments. And now when I go to the grocery store, I see this place less as a place of transience but a museum for these ordinary objects. ■

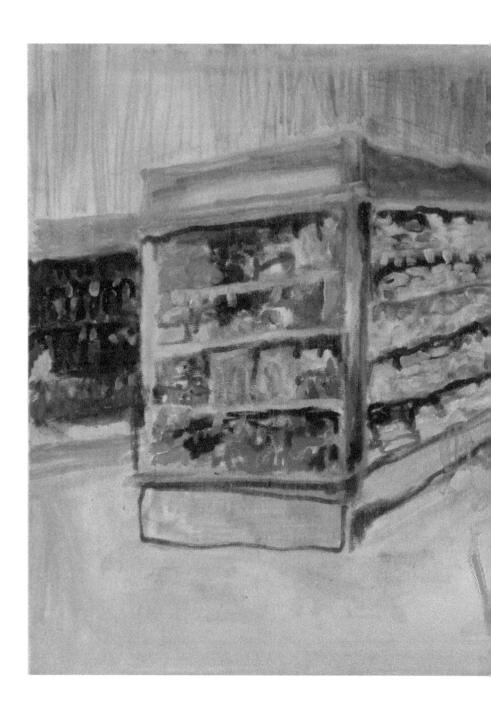

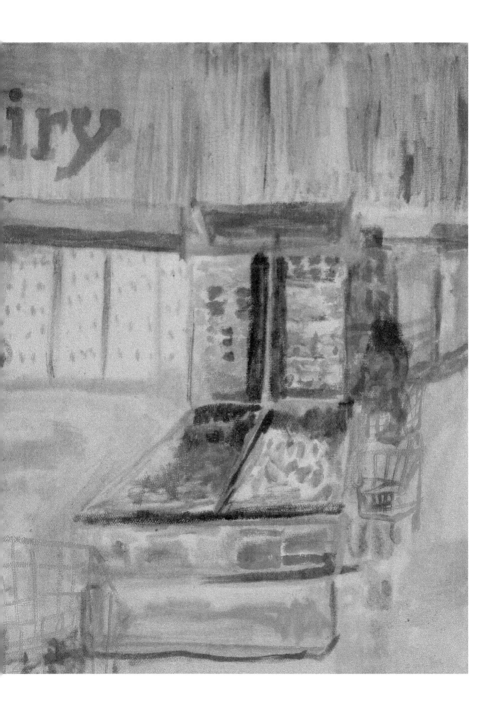

# Background Reading

Odell, Jenny. *How to Do Nothing: Resisting the Attention Economy.* Brooklyn, NY: Melville House, 2019.

Kimmerer, Robin Wall. *Braiding Sweetgrass: Indigenous Wisdom, Scientific Knowledge and the Teachings of Plants.* Minneapolis, MN: Milkweed Editions, 2013.

Tolentino, Jia. *Trick Mirror: Reflections on Self-Delusion.* New York: Random House, 2019.

Kaprow, Allan, and Jeff Kelley. *Essays on the Blurring of Art and Life, Manifesto.* University of California Press, 1996.

Kaprow, Allan, and Jeff Kelley. *Essays on the Blurring of Art and Life, The Real Experiment (1983).* University of California Press, 1996.

Kaprow, Allan, and Jeff Kelley. *Essays on the Blurring of Art and Life, Performing Life (1979).* University of California Press, 1996.

July, Miranda, and Brigitte Sire. *It Chooses You.* Canongate, 2012.

Sagmeister, Stefan, et al. *Things I Have Learned in My Life so Far.* Abrams, 2013.

What are you Looking at?

# Acknowledgments

Thank you to Stephanie Rowden, Jim Cogswell, and Megan Freund for your project oversight and insight.

Thank you to Rebekah Modrak for your guidance and wisdom. Thank you for the cups of tea and listening ears.

Thank you to Stamps and ArtsEngine for funding this project.

Thank you to Miriam Siegel for documenting *Returning Red Solo.*

Thank you to Alex Snow for documenting *Artist-in-Residence.*

Thank you Cynthia Greig for telling me about kintsugi and that my cups follow the tradition.

Thank you Hena Patel, Director of Meijer on Jackson Rd. for accepting my residency proposal.

Thank you to my roommates Katie Seguin and Madalyn Osbourne for your patience when my stuff is all over the house and for your listening ears and copy-editing eyes!

Thank you to my parents and siblings for your love and support always!

My dream dinner party guest list includes Jenny Odell, Jia Tolentino, Robin Wall Kimmerer, Stefan Sagmeister, Allan Kaprow, and Miranda July. Thanks for doing nothing directly for me, but sharing your lives and work so that I learn from everything.

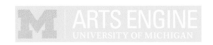

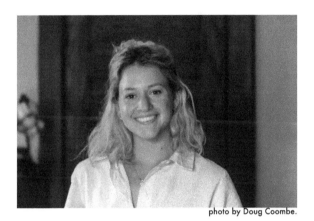

photo by Doug Coombe.

**Erin Wakeland** is a 2020 graduate of the
University of Michigan. This is her integra-
tive project for the Penny W. Stamps BFA
program. She was the first recipient of the Big
Idea Award upon graduation. She enjoys a lot
of things. Some more than others.

erinraywakeland.com

# What are you Looking at?

CPSIA information can be obtained
at www.ICGtesting.com
Printed in the USA
BVHW012138060123
655793BV00027B/398